"I woke up like this!"

We all wish we could wake up looking like something out of a Hollywood movie, don't we? We wish we had flushed, glowing skin, full lips, a great glossy mane of locks, and the youthfulness of a 21 year old. In order to achieve this as we get older, we use a mountain of beauty products and cosmetics, and over those years, these beauty items can have quite the opposite effect.

As well as being costly, a lot of beauty cosmetics these days contain ingredients that aren't exactly great for your skin. What you may find is that a moisturiser may give you moisturising properties, but at the same time, it could contain alcohol to create the fragrance. This alcohol would then dry your skin out, giving you a different problem from the one you started with.

You treat this new dryness with a brand new beauty product, which again may contain another ingredient such as Hydroquinine, which is used to lighten the skin, and this has been linked to problematic reproductive systems, and an increase in various cancers.

Sometimes, it pays to go back to basics when it comes to your beauty regime. There are so many ingredients found in common cosmetics that are not considered safe for your skin, and the question you need to ask yourself is this - if you're not happy eating the ingredient, why would you try to nourish your skin with it?

Mascara and eyedrops, for example, has been known to contain mercury which has been linked to brain impairment. Lead is another carcinogen, show to be linked to increased cancer risks, and is often found in things such as hair dye and lipsticks. Although not commonly listed as an ingredient, which means you won't be able to spot it, it is a regular contaminant of these beauty products and you should therefore be mindful of it.

When you are using DIY beauty recipes to create your own cosmetics and beauty items from home, you are eliminating the risks of doing more harm to your body and skin than good. Why would you use a chemical sunscreen that contains Oxybenzone, something that has been linked to cell damage, low birth weight, disruption of hormones, and even allergies, when you could be using an all-natural sunscreen made with ingredients that offer the properties you need without injecting any bad stuff into it?

For every bad ingredient in the beauty world, there is an all-natural approach around it, as shown by the recipes in this book. So to save your skin, and give you years of youthfulness ahead of you, check out some of these. From toners to shampoos, shower gels to antiperspirant, toothpastes to moisturisers, there's a DIY beauty recipe for everything, and with a dedicated chapter to even the most problematic of skin complaints - eczema, psoriasis, rosacea, and more, you might wonder why you never tried it before!

DIY Beauty Recipes - Specialist Skin   4

1 - Eczema Skin Rub   5

2 - Psoriasis Aloe Vera & Lemon Juice Mask   6

3 - Acne Watermelon & Banana Cocktail   7

4 - Scar-Busting Beauty Balm   8

5 - Sugar, Olive Oil & Lemon Juice Stretch Mark Scrub   9

6 - Coffee Cellulite Scrub   10

7 - Honey Bath Milk for Sunburned Skin   11

8 - Beeswax Body Butter   12

DIY Beauty Recipes - Face   13

1 - Anti-Ageing Facial Serum   14

2 - Yogurt & Honey Face Pack   15

3 - Oil Cleansing Face Treatment   16

4 - Lavender & Orange Lip Balm   17

5 - Banana & Vitamin E Eye Balm   18

6 - Herbal Facial Steam   19

7 - Manly Cucumber Mask (For Men)   20

8 - Rosacea Redness Reducer   21

9 - Nighttime Anti-Wrinkle Serum   22

10 - Mint & Honey Dark Circle Reducer   23

11 - DIY Teeth Whitener   24

12 - Good Morning Moisturiser   25

13 - Cucumber Face Mist   26

14 - Anti-Ageing Face Toner   27

Five Minute Wonders!   28

DIY Beauty Recipes - Hair   30

1 - Fennel Hair Tonic   31

2 - Peppermint & Rosemary Hair Wash   32

3 - Olive Oil & Honey Hair Mask   33

4 - Baking Soda Buildup Buster   34

5 - Banana & Coconut Oil Smoothie   35

6 - Avocado, Banana & Coconut Milk Hair Conditioner   36

7 - Shea Butter, Aloe Vera & Coconut Oil Curl Enhancer   37

8 - Salty-Sea Spray   38

9 - Avocado, Banana & Coconut Milk Hair Conditioner   39

10 - Homemade Healthy Hairspray   40

DIY Beauty Recipes - Body   41

1 - Silky Smooth Legs in a Bottle   42

2 - Green Tea Exfoliating Scrub   43

3 - Argan Oil & Frankincense Body Moisturiser   44

4 - Mint & Aloe Vera Cooling Balm   45

5 - Egg White, Honey & Green Tea Firming Paste   46

6 - DIY Hair Minimising Lotion   47

7 - DIY Anti-Perspirant   48

9 - Sunbaked Fake Tan   49

10 - Vanilla Bean Body Butter   50

DIY Beauty Recipes - Hands & Feet   51

Final Advice & Warnings   54

DIY Beauty Recipes - Specialist Skin

DIY beauty recipes are a great idea for specialist skin, when everything else you've tried has either not worked, agitated the problem further or proved too messy / greasy / flaky to bother with.

Very often, making your own skin care treatment is a last resort, but it should be your first port of call when you have a skin problem. There is a reason some of these recipes have been around for hundreds, and in some cases thousands, of years.

With all-natural ingredients, not only are you ensuring that your skin is healthy, with no unnecessary ingredients clogging up pores or causing more harm than good, but you are creating a range of beauty products that are even safe for your kids to use. Don't they deserve the very best?

You will spend far too many dollars over your lifetime on **this** cream that gets rid of wrinkles, or **that** great gel that combats cellulite, when all the answers have been in your very kitchen the whole time. Did you know that oatmeal or sugar makes a great ingredient for a completely personalised body scrub that smells exactly the way you want it to?

Plus, making your own is super cheap. Why spend $20 on an exfoliating scrub, when you could make something that does the job a thousand times better and costs just a fraction of the price?

So, whether it's eczema that is getting you down, or stretch marks stopping you from being bikini-ready this summer, you need to take a peek at the DIY beauty recipes that actually do the job better than most commercially sold products, and cost less than what you'd spend on an ice cream!

1 - Eczema Skin Rub

Great For: Itchy, irritated skin, eczema, related symptoms

Ingredients:
- 2 tbsp coconut oil
- 3-5 drops essential oil

How-to:
- If coconut oil is solid, warm it in the microwave for 10-15 seconds
- Add drops of essential oil
- Allow to cool to room temperate in small container
- Place in fridge to allow it to become firm

To use:
When you spot your eczema flaring up, use this moisturising rub to soothe away the irritation. The rub can be used when required, or as an all-over body moisturiser to keep your skin soft, and you can make as much or as little as you want. Place the small amount mentioned above in a small, empty lip-balm container with a lid, or in a bigger tub that can be sealed.

Why:
Coconut oil is full of goodness that your skin is crying out for when you're having an eczema flare up. Not only is have antibacterial properties, but also antioxidant, antifungal, and anti-microbial to ensure that your skin is not only well hydrated and moisturised, but clear from gunk and product or dirt buildup. Dirty skin is not good for eczema sufferers.

You can use a wide range of essential oils along with your coconut oil, and you will find that these will make a great addition to your beauty balm:

Lavender - Offers same antibacterial, anti-fungal, and antiseptic properties as the coconut oil, and also helps to moisturise and calm the irritated area. It can help to speed up the healing process, and in some cases, can also help with scarring.

Tea Tree - Antiviral and anti-inflammatory properties are added to the mix with Tea Tree oil and has a lovely smell that proves to be very refreshing on a hot summer's day.

Geranium - Has been shown to kill skin germs, plus it offers a really beautiful, feminine, and upbeat scent.

Thyme - Another energising essential oil offering great calming, cleansing and antibacterial properties.

You may also want to consider - Frankincense, Melrose, and Cedarwood.

2 - Psoriasis Aloe Vera & Lemon Juice Mask

Great For: Itchy, irritated skin, psoriasis, related symptoms

Ingredients:
- 2 Aloe Vera leaves
- Half a lemon

How-to:
- Cut your Aloe Vera leaves, slide it open, and squeeze out the pulp inside
- Cut your lemon in two, and squeeze one-half into a bowl
- Combine the two ingredients in a blender until created into a paste

To use:
Make as much or as little as you need - a small lip-balm sized container is perfect for handbag use when your psoriasis symptoms are at their worst, or you could make a larger tub to use all over your body, arms or legs.

Smear over affected areas, and leave for as long as you can. Rinse off in the shower, and follow with a super conditioning DIY body moisturiser.

Why:
Aloe Vera has been used in cosmetics and medicines for years. In fact, the positive properties go as far back as ancient times, and with a whole range of positive side effects, it's no wonder it's very commonly used in many commercially manufactured beauty products today.

It's calming properties are what makes it so great for psoriasis, and when used on the face, it can also help to remove blemishes and imperfections - it could even have reduce the appearance of scars and stretch marks.

When you mix the Aloe Vera with the lemon in this DIY beauty recipe, you are using the antibacterial and nutritional properties of the citrus fruit to work a bit of extra magic, but it also prevents the Aloe Vera gel from going brown if you're planning on storing it for a little while.

One of the best treatment plans for psoriasis is a very good, hydrating moisturiser, and that's just what you'll get from the gel of the Aloe Vera plant. It contains a high water content, giving your skin the extra boost it needs, and in studies performed on both men and women, Aloe Vera gel helped to clear up symptoms within four weeks in the majority of cases.

3 - Acne Watermelon & Banana Cocktail

Great For: Acne-prone skin - helps to alleviate zits, and prevent further ones!

Ingredients:
- 1 tsp watermelon juice
- 1 tsp mashed banana

How-to:
- Mash the bank with the watermelon juice with a fork until smooth enough to apply as a paste

To use:
When you are suffering from particularly nasty breakouts, or you just want to prevent any further ones, this Watermelon & Banana Cocktail is a great DIY beauty recipe to help combat acne. Simply apply to the affected areas when you are showing symptoms or have some free time, leave for 15-20 minutes, and then rinse off with lukewarm water. Remember to dab dry with a towel, and not rub!

You can repeat this as often as required.

Why:

We'll start with the watermelon - this fruit contains a massive amount of water which will not only rehydrate the skin, but also help to detox it, cleansing it from the toxins, dirt, and buildup that can lead to those dreaded zits. You should think of it like an oil fee moisturiser.

The banana, on the other hand, contains a bunch of B-vitamins (B2, B6, and B12), and these help to keep the redness and inflammation down, as well as moisturising your skin and working hard to keep it soft and supple.

4 - Scar-Busting Beauty Balm

Great For: Reducing the appearance of scars (and stretch marks), and as an all-around great moisturiser for the body and face

Ingredients:
- 1 oz coconut oil
- 10 drops Geranium essential oil
- 8 drops Lemongrass essential oil
- 6 drops Lavender essential oil
- 3 drops Frankincense essential oil
- 3 drops Melrose essential oil

How-to:
- Warm the coconut oil in a double boiler
- Pour into glass jar and allow to cool (Until it is warm, not hot)
- Add all essential oils and stir well

To use:
Twice per day, rub the Scar-Busting Beauty Balm to the scarred areas of the body and allow the body to absorb.

Why:
We already know that coconut oil is great for your skin, but the essential oils contained within this great scar-reducing beauty balm help to create a recipe that not only leaves the skin well-nourished, moisturised and well-hydrated, but also brings a whole bunch of other health benefits.

Geranium has a beautiful, floral scent, and also works as an astringent as well as having antibacterial properties, so not only will it help fight infections, but can also speed up the healing process of cuts, grazes, abrasions and more. By rubbing this essential oil into the skin, you are facilitating blood circulation just under the skin, and this will help to smooth out any problem areas.

Lemongrass offers a number of the same skin benefits and has also been shown to help with cellulite among a number of other skin complaints. Not just that, but the smell alone helps to fight depression with aromatherapy, and can help to lift your spirits - great for use first thing in the morning!

Frankincense is not just good for your skin either - as well as helping to remove the appearance of scars, stretch marks and cellulite, it can also help to heal wounds faster, work as an excellent antiseptic, has anti-ageing properties (great for more mature skin), and can even help with pain relief too!

5 - Sugar, Olive Oil & Lemon Juice Stretch Mark Scrub

Great For: Stretch marks, improving the appearance of blemished skin, removing age spots. Can also be used to even skin before applying fake tan.

Ingredients:
- 2 parts raw cane sugar
- 1 part olive oil
- 1 - 2 tsp lemon juice

How-to:
- Mix the sugar and olive oil together well
- Add the lemon juice
- Stir until it creates a 'scrub' consistency

To use:
Use this beauty treatment two to three times per week on the affected areas of the body to see a visible improvement of stretch marks, and scars too!

Apply to the skin and massage in well, leave for around 15 minutes, and then rinse off.

(Little tip - apply to your skin when you first get in the shower and rinse off at the end once you've washed your hair, etc.)

Why:
Lemon juice is a natural bleach compound, so if you have any dark areas on your skin, this beauty scrub is the way forward. There is citric acid in the lemon juice which help to promote new, healthy skin growth by getting rid of the old skin cells, and when the juice is mixed with the sugar and olive oil, it not only buffs off all the bad skin, but also improves circulation, much in the same way as a tough exfoliating brush would do.

The lemon juice works to reduce the dark colour of the stretch marks, whereas the sugar helps to exfoliate the skin and promote circulation. The olive oil adds a great, luxury moisturising compound to the ingredient and all together; you have a recipe for success!

6 - Coffee Cellulite Scrub

Great For: Combating cellulite, improving circulation, exfoliating

Ingredients:
- 1 cup of ground coffee
- 3 tbsp sea salt or sugar
- 6 tbsp coconut oil

How-to:
- In a large jar, mix the ground coffee and sugar / salt together
- Melt the coconut oil slightly in the microwave if it is solid
- Leave to cool and add coconut oil to mixture
- Store in a sealable container
-

To use:
Once a week, treat yourself to this luxurious Coffee Cellulite Scrub by massaging it in whilst in the shower, scrubbing with an exfoliating brush, and then rinsing off thoroughly.

Why:
Caffeine is for cellulite was Kryptonite is for Superman! The caffeine present in your coffee scrub does many things to improve the appearance of your dimpled skin, and just one of those is to tighten it. Not just that, but it adds powerful antioxidants to the affected areas, making it well-nourished. When your skin is nutrient rich, it is less likely to suffer from cellulite, stretch marks, and a whole host of other complaints.

The sugar or salt in the DIY beauty recipe gives you a rough compound to give the skin a good rub-down, flaking off old, dead skin cells and encouraging new, healthier ones to grow in its place, while the coconut oil brings something beautifully rich and luxurious to the mixture. After just two times using this, you'll notice the difference on your skin, especially on the areas in which you suffer cellulite.

7 - Honey Bath Milk for Sunburned Skin

Great For: Sunburned skin

Ingredients:
- 2 cups oatmeal (uncooked)
- 1 cup whole milk
- 1 tbsp honey

How-to:
- Pour a warm (not too hot) bath
- Add all ingredients
- Relax and chill out for 30 minutes

To use:

You can use this Honey Bath Milk whenever you need to, and it's not just good for sunburned skin although that's what it is particularly great for.

Why:

The oatmeal may seem a little odd but once you get used to it moving around on the bottom of your bath, you'll start to reap the benefits. It works as a natural exfoliator to your skin, encourage it to shed the dead skin cells and create new, healthy ones. Not just that, it can offer healing properties to the skin, and is great for mini-facials.

The milk, on the other hand, offers a richer tone to your bath, bringing a whole host of benefits plus that fat content, being whole milk. There is plenty of protein in milk, which will nourish your skin cells. Not just that, it has great soothing properties, and also contains plenty of various vitamins, in particular - A, D and E. The honey also offers these nutrients but has actually shown to be a natural antiseptic salve too.

8 - Beeswax Body Butter

Great For: Really keeping dry skin in check, and for keeping your skin SUPER smooth

Ingredients:
- 1 vitamin E gel capsule
- 1/2 tsp of your favourite essential oil
- 2 ounces beeswax
- 1/4 cup coconut oil
- 1/8 cup cocoa butter
- 1/8 cup palm oil
- 1 cup olive oil

How-to:
- Using a double boiler system, heat all ingredients (minus vitamin E gel capsule and essential oil)
- When all has melted, take away from the heat
- Add essential oils and vitamin E capsule (it will melt with the heat)
- Pour into a sealable tub (leftover beauty product tub)

To use:
Lather over dry skin as and when needed. Smells great so perfect for everyday use.

Why:

All of the ingredients you're using here are rich ingredients, which means the finished product is going to be thick, and rich, providing plenty of vitamin and nutrient boosts as it is absorbed by your skin.

Vitamin E, for example, is great for a ride range of skin ailments such as sunburn, anti-ageing, and hydrating. If you add various essential oils, you'll also be bringing more benefits such as:

Tea Tree Oil - Great for burns, scalds, sunburned skin, infections
Citronella - Great for repelling summer bugs
Calendula - Great for dry skin, rashes, diaper rash
Chamomile - Great for PMS

Eucalyptus - Great for when you're bunged up, or you have a headache

DIY Beauty Recipes - Face

Your face is the first thing that people see, so it makes sense to want to keep it in tip-top condition. Whether it's suffering from sun damage during the warmer months or being battered by the rain and snow of the colder ones, it sure deserves some TLC from time to time. What better way to show it some love, than nourishing it and pampering it with some luxurious DIY beauty recipes?

It doesn't matter what you're pulling off the shelves in the drug or beauty store. Shampoo, conditioner, mascara, exfoliant, deodorant… Most of them contain products that are **BAD** for your skin.

Take a regular moisturiser, for example. You might notice something called BHT or BHA in the ingredients list. These are both considered to be harmful to fish and other wildlife, so why are they being used in everyday beauty products? BHA has been linked to cancer on more than one occasion, which definitely makes you question your own beauty regime, doesn't it?

What about your shampoo and conditioner? Can you see an ingredient called TEA, MEA or DEA? These are generally used in products that foam and are creamy in consistency and have once again, been linked to cancer, **and** been shown to be harmful to fish and other wildlife.

Most beauty products now, especially deodorants and body sprays, contain something called paragens, and these have been shown to disrupt the reproductive system in men. Triclosan is another one you'll want to keep an eye out for, and even more so in your toothpaste and deodorants. This one can be a contributor to antibacterial resistance to bacteria which means if you need certain drugs to combat disease and illness in the future, they might not work for you because you have created an immunity to them.

With all-natural, DIY beauty recipes, you can be 100% sure of exactly what you are putting in the products you use on and around your face. You can be completely sure that you aren't going to cause any adverse reactions, or use anything that could cause it more harm than good. Fresh fruit, vegetables, herbs and essential oils - all those minerals and vitamins; they aren't just great for your inner body, they're ideal for using in DIY beauty recipes for skin care you can really rely on.

Whether it's acne or rosacea, wrinkles or lip care, teeth cleaning or anti-ageing, there's something natural for everything.

Just take a peek for yourself…

1 - Anti-Ageing Facial Serum

Great For: Those that want to look more youthful for longer

Ingredients:
- 5 drops each of Frankincense, Myrrh, Lavender, and Rose essential oils
- 3 drops of Helichrysum essential oil (can be left out if not found)
- Enough almond oil to fill a small 5 ml bottle

How-to:
- Get yourself a couple of 5ml bottles with lids
- Mix all ingredients together and transfer to smaller bottles

To use:
Can be used every day as an anti-ageing serum, or for when your skin needs a little pick-me-up.

Ideally, you're going to want to put this on right as you get out of the shower in the morning, or even better before you go to bed at night. It can take a little while for the oily goodness to be absorbed into the skin, and makeup may slide if you try to put it on, on top of the serum.

Why:
Almond oil in beauty and medicine can be dated as far back as Ancient China, and the vitamin E, plus omega-3 fatty acids bring a whole host of rewards - reducing dark circles and under-eye bags, getting rid of fine lines, wrinkles and crow's feet, increasing hydration, and a smoothing effect.

Frankincense essential oil can be used by itself to reduce the appearance of spot breakouts. Just dab a tiny bit right onto the spot, and reduce will be reduced almost instantly, with the entire spot dying down within a few hours rather than days.

Myrrh helps you to get great looking skin too, plus the Helichrysum is awesome for its restorative benefits, so if you've got damaged skin, you should try to hunt this down.

2 - Yogurt & Honey Face Pack

Great For: Firming, wrinkle-busting, fighting acne, fixing dislocations and blemishes, relieving sunburn, toning

Ingredients:
- 4 parts yogurt
- 1 part honey

How-to:
- Mix two ingredients in a bowl, adding more yogurt if consistency is too sticky

To use:
Once a week, use this Yogurt & Honey Face Pack all over your face. Simply apply it, wait for 15-20 minutes, and then rinse off, patting dry with a towel.

Why:
Yogurt has a whole bunch of body benefits and with the proteins, vitamin D, calcium, and probiotics, you know it's going to do a great job. Eating it can do as much good as using it cosmetically, but this face pack is a great instant boost for tired, lacklustre skin.

If you apply this cooling pack straight from the fridge, it can help to fight redness and sunburn, offering a cooling sensation. This also makes it great for acne. The probiotics ensure that your good bacteria flourish, whereas the bad bacteria are fought away by your own boosted immune system and cells.

On top of that, the honey helps to firm and tighten, is packed full of amino acids, vitamins and minerals, and has a great, rich consistency, plus a beautiful smell.

3 - Oil Cleansing Face Treatment

Great For: When your face really needs a good cleanse!

Ingredients:
- 1 part caster oil
- 4 parts extra virgin olive oil
- Few drops Tea Tree oil
- Warm, damp face-wash cloth

How-to:
- Add all ingredients together
- Use ratio of 3 parts caster oil to 1 part olive oil if you have very oily skin
- Use ratio of 1 part caster oil to 3 parts olive oil if you have very dry skin

To use:
You will need to move the mixture into a spray bottle to use. Simply spray the cleanser all over your face, massage into the skin for a few moments using circular motions, and then place the damp, warm washcloth over your face. Sit back and relax for ten minutes before removing the cloth, and gently wiping off any reside with clean water.

Why:

Not only will the olive and caster oil leave your skin feeling supple and smooth, but you'll also be pumping it full of good stuff. Olive oil has no fewer than three antioxidants - vitamin E, polyphenols, and phytosterols. These help to make the skin soft but also help to fight back against ageing, so is perfect for the delicate skin on your face. Plus, it doesn't clog your pores like other cleansing products can, and although thick, is easily absorbed.

Caster oil, on the other hand, can help with problems like warts, athlete's foot, chronic itching, and even boils. It also helps to plump up the skin to avoid fine lines and wrinkles, help fight back against acne, works as a great natural moisturiser, and can even help to fade both scars and stretch marks.

Tea Tree oil helps to bring the cleansing treatment together, giving the skin a flushed look, and giving it a good clean to get rid of product residue.

4 - Lavender & Orange Lip Balm

Great For: Giving you kissably soft lips!

Ingredients:
- 1/4 cup coconut oil
- 3 tbsp beeswax pellets
- 10 drops orange essential oil
- 7 drops lavender essential oil
- 1 vitamin E capsule
- 10 small, empty lip balm tubs or tubes

How-to:
- Melt the coconut oil over medium heat
- Add the beeswax pellets
- Take off heat before adding both essential oils
- Poke hole in vitamin E capsule and pour into mixture
- Pour into containers and allow to cool (or place in fridge on a tray)

To use:
Use this every day to prevent chapped lips, or whenever needed.

Why:

For years, orange essential oil has been used to treat and heal, so it's hardly surprising that it should work on chapped or dried lips. Plus, here's a little freebie trick - add a touch of cinnamon to the mixture as you are melting it together, and it makes for great homemade lip balm for Christmas gifts! You could even consider adding chocolate too.

As well as being an anti-inflammatory, orange is an antiseptic, fights back against cancer with powerful antioxidants, and is packed full of vitamin C, meaning you have something that will really fight back against the elements. Plus, the smell will instantly uplift you, and helps to boost blood flow to the area. Following on from this, collagen production is increased so this lip balm could even help you to get fuller, plumper lips too!

5 - Banana & Vitamin E Eye Balm

Great For: When you have puffy / red eyes

Ingredients:
- 1 banana
- 1 / 2 vitamin E capsules

How-to:
- Peel banana
- Mash fruit into a bowl
- Add vitamin E capsules contents

To use:
In the morning when you are getting ready for a big day ahead, use this balm around the eye area when you have been lacking in sleep, crying, or had one too many glasses of wine the night before.

Apply to skin, leave for 10-15 minutes as you are drinking your coffee, and rinse off, dabbing your face dry with a soft towel.

Follow with a good moisturiser, and then your daily makeup.

Why:
Bananas are high in potassium, which has actually been shown to regulate the levels of fluid around the eyes. When you are suffering from puffy eyes, using this for a couple of days can give you dramatically improved results. Long-term use can get rid of puffiness as well as dark circles, and even fine lines and wrinkles, encouraging extra collagen production at the same time.

Vitamin E is already used in a great number of commercially manufactured beauty products, and has been shown to help with a wide range of issues including wrinkles, acne, redness, age spots, collagen production, improving skin tone, and much more!

6 - Herbal Facial Steam

Great For: Improving circulation, improving skin tone, opening pores.

*Shouldn t be used by people with damaged or very dry skin.

Ingredients:
- 1-pint water
- 1/2 cup of dried citrus peel, peppermint leaves, rosemary, lavender flowers, rose petals, chamomile tea (from inside of bag)

How-to:
- Use old fruit peel, let dry overnight, and do the same with lavender flowers, rose petals, etc.
- Boil water
- Add leaves, herbs, etc. and leave to steep for 30 minutes
- Transfer to a large bowl

To use:
Hold face 12 inches above the bowl, using a towel to cover your head. The aim of the game is to use the steam escaping from the bowl to cleanse out your pores, draw out impurities, and rehydrate the skin.

Why:
Water is essential for a healthy body, so anything containing water is just going to add moisture to it. The steam will hit your face and turn back into water (which is why your face feels so damp after using a steam bath), and gives it more hydration, which normally solves a whole bunch of problems.

The steam also helps to draw out impurities from the skin, so any product residue or gunk will be persuaded to come out of the crevices, giving you a real deep clean, and the various herbs bring homeopathic properties to the mix, which have proven themselves for thousands of years, to greatly improve a wide range of issues.

7 - Manly Cucumber Mask (For Men)

Great For: When the fella in your life could do with a good face mask…

Ingredients:
- 1 tbsp full-fat Greek yogurt
- 1/2 cucumber

How-to:
- Remove the peel of the cucumber
- Finely chop cucumber
- Blitz it through a blender until it resembles pulp
- Transfer to a bowl, and spoon in the yogurt

To use:
When you're enjoying a face mask yourself, sit your man down and apply this to his face. You must promise him that you won't take photos and share them over social media. Sit for 10 to 15 minutes, before rinsing off with cool water, and dabbing the skin dry with a towel.

Why:
Although he's too manly for all that face-mask stuff, he won't be able to resist when he feels how soft his skin **COULD** feel after this delicious skin treatment. If you apply this straight from the fridge, it'll have a very calming, soothing effect on the skin, helping with things like sunburn, beard irritation, shaving rash, softening, toning, improving blemished, and more!

It doesn't even matter if he has a beard because, with this great face mask, the yogurt will work its magic on that too, softening the hair and making it much nicer to kiss him.

Cucumber brings with it a whole bunch of skin positives, and just one of them is the water content it holds. It's made up of mostly water so by applying those cucumber slices to your eyes; you are massively hydrating them which in turn can help with puffiness, redness, and even irritation.

The slight bleaching agent it contains will help to even out skin tone, making it great for both men and women, and can even help reduce sun damage, making it a perfect cooling treat for a hot summers day!

8 - Rosacea Redness Reducer

Great For: Red spots, blotchy skin, red and bumpy symptoms of rosacea

Ingredients:
- 1 cup Green Tea
- 1 tsp honey
- 1 tbsp apple cider vinegar
- 2 tbsp plain yogurt (unsweetened)
- 1 - 2 tbsp dry oatmeal

How-to:
- Add oatmeal, honey, apple cider vinegar and yogurt to a blender and blitz until smooth
- Transfer to large bowl
- Add 3 tablespoons Green Tea and mix well
- Continue to add tea slowly, one tablespoon at a time, until it has created a thick paste

To use:
Apply this redness-reducing paste to clean and dry skin, and leave for around 15-20 minutes. Using a cool, damp cloth, wipe off the paste and then rinse your face well with cool water. Pat dry with a towel, before using a natural, light moisturiser.

Why:
You know how you can clean things with vinegar? Well, you can even clean your skin with vinegar, although we wouldn't recommend it neat.

Diluting apple cider vinegar in your DIY beauty recipe is a great idea for many reasons. Firstly, it gives you the chance to give your skin that deep-clean we keep talking about, but on top of that, it can work to eradicate age spots by evening out the skin tone, can help to get rid of acne and little zits by clearing out all the bad stuff that causes them, and it even helps to get rid of that excess oil, making it great to use before summer-day makeup.

9 - Nighttime Anti-Wrinkle Serum

Great For: Getting rid of those pesky wrinkles, serious nourishment of the skin

Ingredients:
- 2 drops Patchouli essential oil
- 3 drops Lemon essential oil
- 5 drops Rose essential oil
- 1 Evening Primrose capsule
- 1 tbsp hazelnut oil (or almond oil)

How-to:
- Mix all ingredients together in a glass bowl
- Can be saved in an airport, sealable container for up to one week

To use:

Use a cotton wool ball to soak in the serum and rub over the skin on your face, after you have cleansed and toned before bed. Allow the serum to work its magic, and rinse thoroughly in the morning when you get up.

Why:

For some, Evening primrose oil is one of the best things to sort the skin out, whether it's acne and spots or wrinkles and age spots. It can also be used anywhere on the body, making it also great for nourishing your hands and feet.

The oil contained within the seeds is light and easily absorbed by your body, giving it extra moisturising power when it needs it the most. Not only that, but when you massage it gently into the skin in circular motions, you are encouraging blood flow and circulation, which means extra nutrients and hydrations get to it from the inside - out. When you eat healthier, your skin will glow!

10 - Mint & Honey Dark Circle Reducer

Great For: When you've partying too long and your eyes are starting to show with heavy, dark under-eye circles

Ingredients:
- Mint leaves
- 1 tbsp honey
- 1 tbsp almond oil

How-to:
- Using a pestle and mortar (or a blender), crush the mint leaves until they form an almost paste like consistency
- Add the honey and almond oil
- Leave to steep overnight

To use:
You can apply this with your fingers or a cotton wool ball to the area underneath the eye before bed. You can also apply it in the morning, but remember it may take a little while to be absorbed into your skin, so makeup may slide. Use light motions starting from your nose, moving in a curved shape following the curve underneath your eye, towards your hairline and ears to encourage blood flow.

Why:
Mint has a natural cooling action on the body, which makes it great used in things such as aftersun, cooling moisturisers, and soothing gels. Haven't you noticed that a lot of leg and foot creams will contain peppermint?

It will cool down the area under your eyes, reducing fluid retention, and encouraging hydration and rejuvenation of new cells. Plus the honey and almond oil create a thick, slow-absorbed moisturiser that will pump your skin full of omega-3 fatty acids, proteins, and plenty more great minerals and vitamins.

11 - DIY Teeth Whitener

Great For: Whitening your teeth to a Hollywood dazzler from the comfort of your own home!

Ingredients:
- 1 tsp baking soda
- 1 tsp hydrogen peroxide (3% - food grade)
- 3-5 drops Peppermint essential oil

How-to:
- Mix the baking soda, hydrogen peroxide, and peppermint essential oils in a saucer

To use:
Dip your wet toothbrush into the mixture and rub over your teeth, in the same way as you would use 'regular' commercially manufactured toothpaste. Use for two minutes, and then repeat the procedure with your regular toothbrush.

Use once / twice per week only. Overuse can lead to sensitivity, whitening of the gums, and pain.

Why:
Baking soda is just one of those things that clean stuff - do you not remember your Grandmother always using it for this or that? Well, it turns out that when you mix it with hydrogen peroxide, you have the basic ingredients for what goes into most other expensive whitening treatments.

12 - Good Morning Moisturiser

Great For: Giving your skin a great kick-start to the day!

Ingredients:
- 1/2 cup Sea Buckthorn
- 1 vitamin E capsule
- 10-15 drops Grapefruit essential oil

How-to:
- Heat the Sea Blackthorn slightly in a double boiler
- Add the contents of the vitamin E capsule
- Stir in the essential oil
- Leave to cool before transferring to an airport, sealable container, and placing in the fridge overnight.

To use:
Use this great morning moisturiser every morning after you cleanse and before you put your makeup on. It's best to do this right after you get out of the shower to give it time to absorb into your skin before you put your makeup on.

Why:
Grapefruit is a very underrated essential oil, and not only does it have the power to wake up your mind first thing in the morning (grapefruit shower gel always works well), but it has also been linked to weight loss, plus a variety of other body benefits.

It can help to clear up acne, with its antiseptic and disinfectant properties, and it also helps to improve lymphatic function. Not just that, but studies have shown it to be particularly beneficial to those that suffer from oily skin, and it also gives it a lovely, refreshing feeling - as though it has had a great spring clean!

The Sea Buckthorn (check out health food stores - most people have never heard of it!) also brings a great variety of positives to the table - vitamins A, C and E, for example, which help to increase collagen production and therefore bust blemishes, wrinkles, scars and more, and also fights off inflammation for problematic skin.

13 - Cucumber Face Mist

Great For: Rejuvenating your face on hot summer days

Ingredients:
- 1 tbsp rose water
- 1 cucumber
- 1 tsp lemon juice
- 1 tsp Aloe Vera gel

How-to:
- Chop & blitz cucumber in a blender
- Strain cucumber and add rest of ingredients to juice left in the bowl
- Stir the mix well
- Blend for one minute longer
- Pour into spray bottle

To use:

On hot days, or when your skin feels tired or dry, lightly spray this Cucumber Face Mist over your face, neck and shoulders.

Why:

Cucumber has a very cooling effect to it, which is why it's so great for deflating puffy eyes, and for reducing redness too. When you re having a flustered, hard day, spray this over your face for instant hydration and refreshment. Keep it in the fridge for an added boost!

14 - Anti-Ageing Face Toner

Great For: All-round nourishment and TLC for normal skin

Ingredients:
- 100ml rose water
- 2 drops Geranium essential oil
- 2 drops Vetiver essential oil

How-to:
- Mix all three ingredients well and transfer to a spray bottle

To use:
Keep this in the fridge and use in the place of your regular facial toner after cleansing, and before moisturising.

Why:
Rose water has been shown for years to be very beneficial to the skin, and with the right combination of essential oils, you'll find a whole bunch of benefits to reap. This face toner will not only moisturise your skin, but will also nourish it, hydrate it, reduce any blemishes or scars, healing sore or broken skin, slow down and reduce the effects of ageing, improve your skin tone, and reduce dryness.

Impressive, right?

Five Minute Wonders!

If you only have five minutes to spare, you can still use a massive variety of DIY beauty recipes that only have one or two easy-to-find ingredients to give your face a little extra TLC.

Take a peek at some of these little five-minute wonders to revitalise and jazz up your beauty regime for better skin, improved acne, and more:

1 - Witch Hazel

Every home should have Witch Hazel because of the great, all-round qualities it has to offer. It's

been used in medicine for years, and there's a good reason for that. It's a natural astringent to start with, and can be used to get rid of too much oil, as well as cleaning out the pores.

Witch Hazel gel is easy to pick up, and when applied to the skin with a cotton wool ball, will not only cleanse the skin, but also get rid of any redness, with the cooling properties it also has. Plus, the astringent makes it great for helping to clear up bad acne breakouts, and it has also been shown to help reduce the appearance of bruises and stretch marks.

2 - Vitamin E Capsules

You know those vitamins and minerals you buy from the health food store, take for a couple of days, and then forget to take again? Well, many of these can be used as DIY beauty treatments, and one classic example is the humble vitamin E capsule.

You'll have noticed that these are in many of the recipes you'll find within this book, and there's a really good reason for that - it has so many skin-boosting properties, even the cosmetic manufacturers are jumping in on the bandwagon.

Pop open one of your capsules and use your finger to lightly massage the oil into the area underneath your eyes. It helps to get rid of puffiness, dark circles, and even fluid retention.

Evening Primrose capsules are also great for this, and when applied to really dry skin, can have it cleared up and back to completely moisturised in no time at all. Oh, and it can even help to clear spots up faster, so if you need to get picture-perfect ready in time for a big event, a couple of dabs of this magical oil and you'll be red-free in no time.

3 - Peppermint Oil

If you want plumper lips, dab some peppermint oil on them before you apply your lip gloss. If you have a massive red spot, pop some toothpaste or peppermint oil on it to help reduce redness and the swelling. If you have tried, grey looking skin, use a few drops of peppermint oil in your daily moisturiser to help rejuvenate it and get the blood pumping again.

In short, peppermint, and mint, in general, is really good to use in your beauty regime, and at the very least, you should have some of this essential oil in your medicine cupboard to help solve a mountain of problems!

4 - Vaseline & Sugar

A combination of these two mixed together to form a grainy paste is the perfect trick to getting a kissably soft, lipstick-ready pout. Get yourself a toothbrush that you'll use just for this, and apply the mixture to your lips in a circular motion. Massage in for a few minutes before rinsing off and following with a great, moisturising lip balm. Perfect smackers in no time!

5 - Water & Green Tea

Have you run out of toner? Don't despair, make yourself a cup of green tea, let it cool down and use it in the place of your regular toner. It offers all the same properties that most toners offer, except it'll cost you a lot less, and do a better job.

DIY Beauty Recipes - Hair

Over the years, your hair may have suffered at the hands of over-bleaching, over-dyeing, straightening, curling, hair-spraying, back-combing, colour build-up, over-styling, sun damage and a whole load more besides.

Sometimes, it pays to go back to basics and using an all-natural approach to getting your hair back into tip top condition is a great idea. Luckily for you, there are a whole bunch of DIY beauty recipes perfectly designed to treat even the very worst of hair problems.

Even if you don't have years of hair abuse behind you, a 100% natural approach to taking care of your hair is smart, giving you plenty of added protection against future damage, including just being sat out in the glorious sun… Or the miserable rain and cold!

There are more than a few ingredients you'll find around your kitchen to help combat a whole host of hair quandaries. Beer, for example, is not just great for a boozy night out, but is also packed full of vitamins and proteins, all of which can help contribute to healthy hair. With reports of more body, thicker, and fuller hair, perhaps it's time you washed with it, rather than washed it down.

The egg is another classic example of a simple kitchen ingredient you can use within your beauty regime, making your hair shiny and glossy. Once again, pumping it full of proteins, eggs encourage your locks to grow stronger, thicker, and better looking.

In fact, there are so many natural ingredients that can be used to create your own beauty range at home. Not only will you be saving your hair and the environment, you'll also be saving yourself a small fortune too. If only you knew that an olive oil and honey mask could do twice the work that your regular conditioner could achieve… And a bottle of these for your DIY beauty recipes will last you FOREVER!

Whether it's oily hair, dandruff, curly hair or just a bit of extra hydration, there's a DIY beauty recipe for everything.

Just take a peek and see…

1 - Fennel Hair Tonic

Great For: Dandruff, itchy scalp, hair breakage, and shedding.

Ingredients:
- 2 tbsp vegetable glycerin
- 1/4 cup raw apple cider vinegar
- 1 cup filtered water
- 1 tbsp fennel seeds

How-to:
- Bring water to boil in small pan, over high heat
- Crush seeds with back of a spoon (or pestle and mortar)
- Pour boiling water over the seeds
- Add remainder of ingredients
- Sit for 30-45 minutes
- Sieve into a glass jar

To use:

Apply plenty of your Fennel Hair Tonic to your hair and scalp, massage in, and leave for as long as possible (minimum of 5-10 minutes) before rinsing out thoroughly.

Why:

This aromatic herb might be closely related to parsley, but fennel is great for restoring the skin's natural balance, combating excess oil, and soothing dry or irritated skin. Fennell helps the body to create iron for more red blood cells, improving circulation. Some studies have shown it to help with hair loss.

2 - Peppermint & Rosemary Hair Wash

Great For: Oily scalp, dandruff, no-chemical approach

Ingredients:
- 1/2 cup filtered water
- 1/2 cup Castile soap (or another olive oil-based soap)
- 2 drops Peppermint essential oil
- 16 drops Rosemary essential oil

How-to:
- Add castile soap to container
- Pour in Rosemary and Peppermint essential oils
- Add filtered water
- Shake well
- Pour into flip-top container

To use:

Apply to wet hair and lather up. Leave for a few minutes before rinsing. Follow with a gentle conditioning rinse or tonic.

Why:

If you're looking for a no-chemical approach to your hair, perhaps because of over-treatment or colouring, an all-natural shampoo or hair wash is the way forward. Essential oils are great for nourishing as well as cleansing, and both Rosemary and Peppermint have been shown to sort out an oily scalp and dandruff. Plus, they smell beautiful together giving you an added bonus.

You could also consider substituting the Rosemary and Peppermint essential oils for Lavender, Lemon, and even Cypress oils to help combat oily hair.

3 - Olive Oil & Honey Hair Mask

Great For: Hair in dire need of hydration and TLC, over-bleached hair, sun-damaged hair

Ingredients:
- 2 tbsp honey
- 4 tbsp olive oil

How-to:
- Heat olive oil in the microwave for approx. 20-30 seconds
- Add honey and mix well

To use:
Apply to wet hair, cover with a shower cap, and leave for 20-30 minutes (or longer if you can).

Why:

The honey is full of antioxidants, plus its what nature likes to call a 'natural humectant', which

means it will attract moisture. It's also packed full of nutrients to feed the hair and encourage growth.

Olive oil adds moisture to the hair, and also helps to promote hair growth, plus a healthy scalp, and can even help repair damaged hair shafts.

4 - Baking Soda Buildup Buster

Great For: For when your hair has product buildup

Ingredients:
- 1 / 2 tbsp baking soda
- 1 tbsp water

How-to:
- Mix the baking soda and water together until you have formed a thick paste.

To use:
This should be applied to damp hair, left for around fifteen minutes, then rinsed out thoroughly, and shampooed twice. If you have heavy buildup, you can do this every two weeks.

Why:

Nothing gets rid of dirt and grime quite like baking soda, so it's not advisable to use this on really dry hair. Sodium bicarbonate, the key ingredient in baking soda, cuts through anything acidic, so it won't take long to strip the hair back down to its natural beauty.

Do not repeat this more regularly than every two weeks to avoid damaging your hair.

5 - Banana & Coconut Oil Smoothie

Great For: Hair in dire need of hydration and TLC, over-bleached hair, sun-damaged hair

Ingredients:
- 1 banana
- 1 tbsp coconut oil

How-to:
- If the coconut oil is solid, warm it slightly in microwave
- Mash up a banana
- Mix the two ingredients together

To use:
You can use this just where you need it - on the ends or all over your hair. Once you have mixed the two ingredients into something that resembles a smoothie, massage into either damp or dry hair (not wet) and leave for 30 minutes before rinsing out thoroughly, and shampooing twice.

Why:
The banana is jam-packed full of nutrients, giving your hair hydration and food. This will help to repair damaged hair, plus give encourage new growth, stronger and healthier than it was before.
The coconut oil is a very heavy compound, so it really gets deep into the hair strands, taking the nutrients even further.

6 - Avocado, Banana & Coconut Milk Hair Conditioner

Great For: Dry, damaged hair that lacks volume and glossiness, hair loss

Ingredients:
- 1 ripe banana
- 1 - 2 tbsp avocado
- 3-4 tbsp coconut milk

How-to:
- Heat olive oil in the microwave for approx. 20-30 seconds
- Add honey and mix well

To use:
Add to dry hair, leave for 30 minutes, rinse out thoroughly and shampoo. It might be wise to avoid conditioner if you have used this mask to prevent really oily or greasy hair.

Why:
The good news about this DIY beauty recipe is that you can mix up the ingredients to suit you. Banana has been shown to help with things like dandruff, split ends, boosting elasticity, and even shine. You could add more avocado if you wanted - it's been shown to help with hair loss, encourage hair growth, improving the condition, and boosting elasticity. The coconut milk has a high fat content so pumps your locks full of goodness and is also packed with vitamin E - the one of the important vitamins to promote healthy hair.

7 - Shea Butter, Aloe Vera & Coconut Oil Curl Enhancer

Great For: For when your curly hair just won't behave itself! Or for when you have dandruff, dry hair, hair loss, hair thinning

Ingredients:
- 2 tsp Coconut Oil
- 2 tbsp Shea Butter
- 2 tbsp Aloe Vera gel

How-to:
- Mix all ingredients together well
- Put into a sealed container
- Can be kept for up to two weeks

To use:
Every day, twist a very small amount of the curl enhancing balm to the curls of your hair, twisting them around as you go. The balm will help to define the curls, as well as to keep them in place.

Why:
Firstly, this stuff works just like an all-natural curl gel, and can be used daily to help define your hair, as well as nourish it. If you're worried about hair loss, it's also great to use because it contains a natural enzyme that actually encourages the hair to grow. It also helps to get rid of dead skin cells, because of the proteolytic enzymes, and this can help to eradicate dandruff.

8 - Salty-Sea Spray

Great For: Getting beautiful, beach waves on those days when straight hair just won't do!

Ingredients:
- 8 ounces water
- 1 tsp hair gel
- 3 tsp salt

How-to:
- Mix all three ingredients together well in a spray bottle
- Can be kept for 3/4 weeks
- Needs to be shaken before every use

To use:
Spray the hair lightly with the Salty-Sea Spray, while scrunching with your hands. The gel and salt work together to create beachy / Boho waves.

Why:
Sometimes your hair needs a day off, so why not give it just that with this easy to make spray? It works even on greasy / oily day, and when scrunched into the hair and completed with a bandana, beach hat, or even cute, scruffy pigtails, will make the perfect look for a lazy summer's day!

9 - Avocado, Banana & Coconut Milk Hair Conditioner

Great For: Dry, damaged hair that lacks volume and glossiness, hair loss

Ingredients:
- 1 ripe banana
- 1 - 2 tbsp avocado
- 3-4 tbsp coconut milk

How-to:
- Heat olive oil in the microwave for approx. 20-30 seconds
- Add honey and mix well

To use:
Add to dry hair, leave for 30 minutes, rinse out thoroughly and shampoo. It might be wise to avoid conditioner if you have used this mask to prevent really oily or greasy hair.

Why:
The good news about this DIY beauty recipe is that you can mix up the ingredients to suit you. Banana has been shown to help with things like dandruff, split ends, boosting elasticity, and even shine. You could add more avocado if you wanted - it's been shown to help with hair loss, encourage hair growth, improving the condition, and boosting elasticity. The coconut milk has a high fat content so pumps your locks full of goodness and is also packed with vitamin E - the one of the important vitamins to promote healthy hair.

10 - Homemade Healthy Hairspray

Great For: When your hair could do with a little TLC, to avoid alcohol-pumped commercially bought products

Ingredients:
- 1.5 cups boiled or filtered water
- 1 tbsp vodka or other high-proof alcohol
- 2 tbsp white sugar
- 15 drops of your choice of essential oil

How-to:
- You will need to boil your water
- Add the sugar, stirring until dissolved.
- Cool to about room temperature
- Add your choice of booze
- Add your essential oils.

To use:

Pour into a spray bottle and use whenever you would normally use hairspray! It's as simple as that!

Why:

Firstly, you're using all-natural products so you won't have any of that bad product build up.

Secondly, the essential oil you use will change the other properties your hairspray can bring to the table. Basil, for example, can help combat oily hair, and can speed up hair growth. Chamomile is great for fine hair, and not only helps to condition the scalp, but also soothes inflammation, and can help with things such as psoriasis.

DIY Beauty Recipes - Body

It may seem like a lot of hard work, making your own beauty treatments from scratch, but in the long run, not only will you save yourself a small fortune, but you'll be doing your body a massive favour too.

Let's say that the average bottle of good-quality moisturiser will set you back anywhere from $5-$10. You could get some of these ingredients for less than that, and they'll last much longer too.

Not just that, of course, but some of the beauty products you are using could even be causing other problems.

Let's say you use a moisturiser that has Propylene Glycol in the ingredients list. This may help your moisturiser smell nice and spread evenly over your skin, but it's also been shown to cause dry skin and irritation, meaning you'll use more of the stuff to try and combat the problem. When you make your own beauty treatments using ingredients you'd happily put in your mouth, you know you won't be creating your own beauty dilemmas.

There are a lot of beauty products that could actually cause a bunch of other problems too. Anything that contains a petroleum by-product, for example, may leave your skin feeling soft for a while, and work as a great lubricant or base carrier, but over time, it will cause your pores to become clogged.

The molecules that make up petroleum products are too big for your skin to be absorbed, and can lead to issues like acne, uneven skin tone, and more. Why would you still be putting beauty items that contain just that on your skin?

Why not take a peek at these great substitutions for many of the commercially created products you buy? They're cheaper, better for you and bring more benefits than you could think of.

What are you waiting for?

1 - Silky Smooth Legs in a Bottle

Great For: Exfoliating, moisturising, smoothing, to even-out complexion and tone

Ingredients:
- 1 cup sugar
- 2 tbsp lemon juice
- 1/2 cup olive oil
- 5-10 drops essential oil

How-to:
- Grab a large bowl
- Throw all ingredients in
- Mix well
- That's actually how easy it is!

To use:
When you have half an hour spare at the end of a busy week, why not give your legs the treat they deserve, and make use of Silky Smooth Legs in a Bottle. Smother all over the legs just before you get in the shower (whilst standing on a towel), and massage in well - much in the same way as you'd use any body scrub. Leave on for as long as you can, before rinsing off thoroughly in the shower.

Note: This is not one to try in the bath… Unless you want to sit in it.

Why:
The sugar works in two ways in this leg treatment. Firstly, it is rough so when it is applied to the skin and massaged around, it is 'scratching' off the old, dead skin cells. When the skin is massaged, blood is pumped to it, which can improve circulation, and also encourage the growth of fresh new skin cells - stronger and better than the ones before.

The lemon juice works as a natural bleaching agent, so it will help to even out the tone of your legs, as well as getting it ready for all that tanning you're going to want to do this summer. It can help to lighten the skin too if you have any dark patches you'd quite like to get rid of.

The olive oil is a rich, thick ingredient and is full of Omega-3 fatty acids, which the body just loves! This will make sure that your skin is nourished and plumped up, making it less likely for you to suffer from things such as stretch marks, cellulite, or wrinkles.

The essential oil you use is down to you - there are various ones you could use for various reasons. To start with, have a look at some of these:

Carrot Seed essential oil - Great for anti-ageing, fading scars, cell regeneration, and smoothing.
Lemon essential oil - Great scent, also has astringent and antibacterial benefits.
Neroli essential oil - Great for anti-ageing and mature skin, chemical compounds help with skin rejuvenation (citral) and also helps with stretch marks!

2 - Green Tea Exfoliating Scrub

Great For: Great substitute for DIY beauty scrubs that contain coffee, moisturising, softening

Ingredients:
- 1 cup coconut oil
- 2 Green Tea bags
- 2 tsp Green Tea powder
- 1 cup brown sugar

How-to:
- Grab a large bowl
- Mix all ingredients together (empty the teabags into the mix)
- Store in an airtight, sealable container

To use:
Use this Green Tea Exfoliating Scrub whenever you would use a regular exfoliating scrub and not only will you be saving a ton of cash, but you'll be doing your body a whole bunch of favours! Simply apply, massage in, and rinse off in the shower, using an exfoliating glove or mitt.

Why:
Green Tea has so many body-benefits! It has been linked to increased weight loss, better skin, faster-growing hair, improving the digestive tract, and so much more besides. By substituting the coffee / salt / sugar from other scrubs with Green Tea powder, you are adding antioxidants to your recipe, and these have been shown to reduce the chances of cancer.

It's coming up to summer now, so there's never been a better tie to try Green Tea. It has been shown to improve your skin's protection against the sun when used under suncream, so why not give your skin some added protection this year?

3 - Argan Oil & Frankincense Body Moisturiser

Great For: Everyone! Particularly good for very dry skin, problem areas, heels

Ingredients:
- 10 drops Carrot Seed oil
- 10 drops Lavender oil
- 15 drops Frankincense oil
- 2 oz. Argan oil

How-to:
- Mix all ingredients into a bowl
- Pour into a sealable container

To use:
Can be used every day, or just when needed. Simply apply to the skin as you would normally use a moisturiser.

Why:
Argan oil is great for softening skin, and the mixture of essential oils are great for various things, but just the tip of the iceberg are softening, moisturising, antibacterial, anti-fungal, and more.

Rich in fatty acids, carotenes, and vitamin E, Argan oil has recently increased in popularity, and although great for hair, has also shown to be particularly beneficial for dry skin. It can be used, however, by all skin types.

4 - Mint & Aloe Vera Cooling Balm

Great For: Tired legs and body after a long day at work!

Ingredients:
- 5-10 drops Peppermint Essential Oil
- 1/2 cup Aloe Vera gel
- 1/2 cup coconut oil
- 1/4 cup beeswax

How-to:
- Start by grating your beeswax and collecting into a saucepan
- Add the coconut oil and place over low heat until just melted
- Remove from the heat and lightly whisk in the Aloe Vera gel
- Add peppermint essential oil and continue to stir
- Allow to cool for around one hour, and pop in your blender for around 30 seconds until it's fluffy

To use:
Whenever your legs are tired, or your body aches from a heavy day (or night), use the Mint & Aloe Vera Cooling Balm. Ca be used as often as required.

Why:
You'll probably already have noticed that many commercially sold feet and leg cooling lotions

already contain peppermint essential oil, and it is considered to be one of nature's finest coolants. It helps to soothe and calm aching, and tired legs, and has been also been shown to help with restless leg syndrome. It can also help with stinky feet!

5 - Egg White, Honey & Green Tea Firming Paste

Great For: When you really want firm, supple skin all over!

Ingredients:
- 2 egg whites
- 1 - 2 tbsp honey
- 2 tbsp Green Tea

How-to:
- First, steep Green Tea tea bag in hot water until it cools
- Beat two egg whites
- Add honey and cooled Green Tea
- Whisk until a firm, peaked paste

To use:
You can use this paste all over your body, whenever you have the time to use it! Once a week, or once a day - it's up to you! It's all natural, so you can never have too much of it.

Before you have a shower, apply the paste to the areas of the skin you want to firm up, leave for about ten to fifteen minutes and then rinse off thoroughly!

Why:
The caffeine in the Green Tea is what gives this paste the firming qualities it has. Anything containing caffeine will help the skin to spring back to firmness, encouraging tightening and elasticity.

Egg whites, on the other hand, offer proteins to the skin, which make up the building blocks of your cells. The protein helps the cells to grow healthy and strong, and also to rejuvenate.

Smart tip for you - the egg whites help your skin to become more elastic, so when you are preparing your body for pregnancy, it is well worth considering using this firming paste as you are trying to conceive, and throughout the pregnancy!

6 - DIY Hair Minimising Lotion

Great For: When you're really sick of shaving all the time…

Ingredients:
- 4 oz sweet almond oil
- 5 drops lemon essential oil
- 20 drops clary sage essential oil

How-to:
- Mix all three ingredients together in a bowl

To use:
Use this lotion every day for the hair minimising properties with long term use.

Why:
There have been a few reports and old wive's tales over the years that suggest the essential oil clary sage is great for minimising hair growth on the areas on which it is used, and after trawling through various forums on the DIY beauty topic, it would appear that this seems to be true…

You could always try substituting the lemon essential oil for vanilla if you want a sweeter scent, but the lemon ones smell a little like fruity tea and doesn't stick around for too long. Plus the sweet almond oil really nourished your skin, leaving it silky soft and smooth.

7 - DIY Anti-Perspirant

Great For: Taking an all-natural approach to fighting sweat

Ingredients:
- 20-25 drops essential oil - your pick!
- 4 vitamin E capsules
- 15g DE (food grade)
- 15g arrow root powder
- 10g almond oil
- 10g beeswax
- 20g shea butter
- 30g coconut oil

How-to:
- Using a double boiler, melt beeswax, shea butter, and coconut oil
- Take away from heat and leave to cool
- Add remainder of ingredients and whisk vigorously
- Pour into containers and leave to cool overnight

To use:

It may take a couple of attempts, but you're looking for a consistency that is firm yet easy to spread with your fingers, and if you can find empty roll-on sticks, you could use them in the same way.

Why:

All of the ingredients are great for your skin, and you can make your pick of the essential oils to create your very own signature scent… or scents! The vitamin E helps to nourish the armpits, plus the mixture of base oils really moisturise the area. Try it for a few weeks and you'll never go back to your old deodorant ever again!

9 - Sunbaked Fake Tan

Great For: For a sun-kissed glow that won't leave you orange…

Ingredients:
- 16 oz water
- 1 tbsp vanilla extract
- 8 organic black tea bags

How-to:
- Add vanilla extract to water and bring to the boil
- Take off heat, add tea bags, leave to cool for 30 minutes
- Remove tea bags

To use:
Exfoliate first (basic of any great fake tan), and moisturise with a healthy DIY lotion. Using a spray bottle, spritz the fake tan over your body, wait 2 minutes, and then rub in with a fake tan mitt. Leave to dry and repeat. Do this 3/4 times, or until desired brown-ness has been achieved.

Why:
The vanilla extract will make you smell good enough to eat, and the steeped tea bags will create a fake tan spray that will do exactly the same job as those expensive ones you can buy. Plus, you'll be injecting your skin with water which is great to keep it in tip-top condition!

10 - Vanilla Bean Body Butter

Great For: Date night! ;)

Ingredients:
- 1 cup raw cocoa butter
- 1 vanilla bean
- 1/2 cup coconut oil
- 1/2 cup sweet almond oil

How-to:
- Melt the coconut oil and cocoa butter together
- Remove from heat and leave for 30 minutes
- Using a food processor, blitz the vanilla bean
- Add the crushed vanilla bean and sweet almond oil to mixture and stir well
- Transfer to containers and freeze for 30 minutes
- Using food processor, whip until it looks like butter

To use:

If you want to smell good enough to eat, you'll need to use this Vanilla Bean Body Butter in place of your regular moisturiser as you get ready for your date. Smother this luxurious butter all over your body, and let the special recipe do the rest. He'll put putty in your hands.

Why:
Vanilla is a pretty sensual scent so using it in your beauty regime is a recipe for success! He's smelling this luscious scent all over your body, which will baby smooth, evenly toned, and soft enough for him to want to run his hands all over you!

DIY Beauty Recipes - Hands & Feet

Your hands and feet are just important as the rest of your body, but they seem to be the one area we neglect the most. To give your hands a bit of tender loving care, check out some of these amazing DIY beauty recipes that will combat hard skin, age spots, dry skin, bad nails, crappy cuticles, plus a whole bunch more!

1 - Hard Skin Softener

You'll need: Extra virgin olive oil, sea salt, lavender essential oils

If you mix the olive oil and sea salt together, you'll come up with a great beauty scrub that can work a whole world of magic on your feet. Add a few drops of lavender essential oils and it'll not only smell delicious, it helps to heal cracked, dry skin on your feet, and will also offer a calming effect - great after a hard day at work!

All you need to do is rub the Hard Skin Softener over your feet in circular motions, before leaving to soak in for around 15 minutes. Rinse off well, and dab dry, following with a rich moisturiser.

2 - Cuticle Cream

You'll need: 1 tbsp organic beeswax, 2 tbsp organic shea butter, 1 vitamin E capsule, 5 drops orange essential oil, 5 drops lavender essential oil

This one requires some heat, and once you've melted your shea butter and beeswax in a double boiler, you'll need to add the rest of the ingredients and mixing well. Allow to cool and transfer to your container and use whenever your cuticles need a real helping hand. The essential oils will help to keep the area clean and fresh with antifungal and antiseptic properties, plus it'll smell really good and make your hands as soft as anything.

3 - Olive Oil Nail Cream

You'll need: Olive oil! That's really it!

This recipe is a simple one - heat the olive oil up until it is warm to touch and rub into your hands, cuticles and nails at night before you go to bed. For an extra boost, you could even wear your cotton moisturising gloves all night too and give the nourishing treat a chance to get stuck in.

The vitamin E contained in olive oil helps to improve circulation and repair damaged cells, so broken and fragile nails will be strengthened, and they'll grow a bit faster too!

4 - Orange Juice Manicure

You'll need: A couple of oranges.

This one is super-simple - juice your oranges and with the juice, soak your nails in them for at least ten minutes. Why? Well, it's the vitamin C content here - it helps to improve the state of your nails, as well as get rid of any old nail-varnish staining, and kill off any bad bacteria too. Just make sure you use a good moisturiser afterwards - the acid in the fruit can dry your skin out.

5 - Milk & Honey Strengthening Nail Soak

You'll need: 1 tbsp honey, 1/4 cup milk, 2 egg yolks, lightly beaten

Mix all the ingredients together and then soak your nails for about 15 minutes. Rinse your hands off well and you'll notice they are smoother, softer, and evenly toned. Plus, the protein in the egg yolks will help feed your nails, and encourage them to grow stronger and faster.

6 - Watermelon Age Spot Remover

You'll need: A watermelon! (Or fresh watermelon juice / watermelon essential oils)

There are vitamins A, B and C in watermelon, all of which contribute to healthy skin. Age spots are caused by sun damage, and all there of those vitamins can help undo some of that damage. High in moisture and fibre also, use it twice per week for optimal results.

7 - Yogurt Hand Mask

You'll need: Plain yogurt, 5-10 drops essential oil

Plain yogurt works as a great natural mask for the skin on your hands, and when a couple of drops of essential oils are added, give you soft skin that smells great too. Not only will the yogurt mask help to fight age spots, but it will also improve the texture and tone of your skin, giving your hands a more youthful appearance.

8 - Softening Overnight Hand Cream

You'll need: 1/4 cup coconut oil, 1/8 cup cocoa butter, 1/8 cup shea butter, 1 tbsp Aloe Vera gel, 1 tbsp jojoba oil, 10 drops vanilla and fruity essential oil (I like strawberry)

You'll need to melt the shea butter, cocoa butter, and coconut oil together before adding the rest of your ingredients and allowing to cool overnight in the fridge. You'll be glad you did though - apply this hand cream before you go to bed at night, pop a pair of cotton moisturising gloves on over the top, and when you awake, your hands will be so soft, you won't be able to stop touching them.

Nourishing your nails, rejuvenating your skin, and giving your hands a much-needed boost of hydration - that's what you'll get froths softening overnight cream.

9 - Aloe Vera Cooling Foot Spray

You'll need: 5-10 drops peppermint essential oil, 3 tbsp Witch Hazel, 3 tbsp Aloe Vera gel

Add the ingredients, starting with the Aloe Vera gel and ending with the essential oils, and rigorously shake until combined. Store in the fridge for a super-cooling sensation, and use whenever your legs and feet are tired, swollen, or sore. This is also great to use on the arms, and all over the body during the hot summer weather, and the Aloe Vera works great as a soothing aftersun lotion or treatment for sunburn.

10 - Green Tea Soothing Foot Spray

You'll need: 1-2 cups cold water, 2 Green Tea bags

Boil the water with the tea bags in, take off the heat, and leave to cool for a couple of hours. Take the tea bags out, put this soothing tonic into a spray bottle, and store in the fridge until needed.

This is great for cooling down hot and sweaty summer hands, and also for soothing hot and bothered, heavy legs. When you feel uncomfortable in the summer, spray this on your hands and feet for an instant cool down.

11 - Sensual Foot Massage Oil

You'll need: 4 drops lemongrass essential oil, 6 drops peppermint essential oil, 10 drops orange essential oil, 5 tbsp sweet almond oil

Making this is just the perfect excuse to get someone to give you a really good foot massage! If you've ever suffered from sore, stressed, or tired feet, you're going to love the way this feels as it makes its way through your skin, and it can help battle hard skin too!

12 - Refreshing Foot Soak

You'll need: 5 drops peppermint essential oil, 5 drops Tea Tree essential oil, 1 cup Epsom salts

In a plastic basin, add all of the ingredients, swish around, and then rest your weary feet. The Tea Tree oil will get rid of any nasty bugs that shouldn't be there, and the peppermint will help to soothe away those aches and pains with a beautiful cooling sensation. Not just that, but the salts will help to exfoliate any dead skin cells off, and the peppermint will improve circulation and, therefore, nourish the skin.

It would be a shame not to, right?

13 - Male Foot Massage Oil

You'll need: 50 ml sweet almond oil, 6 drops sandalwood essential oil

He'll love you if you give him a massage with this many and sensual foot massage oil. In fact, you could use this all over the body which isn't a bad idea seeing as sandalwood is said to be an aphrodisiac for men...

Final Advice & Warnings

There are a few things you'll need to bear in mind when using some of the ingredients listed in this book of DIY beauty recipes.

Essential oils, for example, are something you'll need to keep your eye on. Make sure that you are using oils that are specifically stated to be safe for use on your skin. You could run the risk of developing a bad reaction if you don't - the exact opposite of what you are trying to achieve.

In fact, make sure that you only ever use ingredients on your skin that specifically stated to be safe for use on your skin.

All of the ingredients listed in this book can be found online, or in health food stores. All of the recipes work out cheaper to buy and make than it is to buy, especially with some of the recipes that you can create in bilk and store for further use. You will also find that many of the ingredients are ones that you'll have already lying around in your kitchen. If the food does you good when you eat it, there's a good chance it will do you good if you use it on your skin.

Never use essential oils undiluted on the skin. They should always be used in a carrier oil or base. This amount should be even less when using the recipe son children.

Always perform an allergy test on the inside of your forearm whenever you are using something you are not sure of. Also, remember that some of the oils stated will contain nuts or nut traces, so if you are allergic to nuts, try to find alternatives. Most of the carrier oils and bases can be substituted for other versions - cocoa butter for shea butter, or olive oil in place of sweet almond oil.

Don't use any essential oils if you are pregnant, and seek advice before trying any of the recipes in this book. There is a whole list of essential oils you should not use when pregnant, and these include many that we have mentioned in this book - cinnamon, chamomile, clary sage, fennel, ginger, jasmine, myrrh, peppermint, rosemary, sage, thyme…

Never store your essential oils in plastic bottles as they can erode and leak. Always be careful when using essential oils on surfaces - it can erode soft surfaces, especially if left uncleaned.